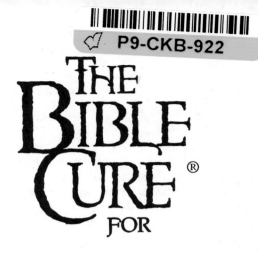

THE BIBLE CURE® FOR

SLEEP DISORDERS

DON COLBERT, M.D.

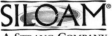

SILOAM®
A STRANG COMPANY

THE BIBLE CURE FOR SLEEP DISORDERS by Don Colbert, M.D.
Published by Siloam
A Strang Company
600 Rinehart Road
Lake Mary, Florida 32746
www.siloam.com

Library of Congress Catalog Card Number: 00-112301
International Standard Book Number: 0-88419-748-4

This book is not intended to provide medical advice
or to take the place of medical advice and treatment
from your personal physician. Readers are advised to
consult their own doctors or other qualified health
professionals regarding the treatment of their
medical problems. Neither the publisher nor the
author takes any responsibility for any possible consequences from any treatment, action or application
of medicine, supplement, herb or preparation to any
person reading or following the information in this
book. If readers are taking prescription medications,
they should consult with their physicians and not
take themselves off of medicines to start supplementation without the proper supervision of a physician.

04 05 06 07   11 10 9 8
Printed in the United States of America

Rest Assured

If sleeping disorders have left you feeling exhausted, depleted and defeated, rest assured that these things are not God's will for you. You can discover real rest and wonderful refreshing in God. The Bible declares, "Jesus said, 'Come to me, all of you who are weary and carry heavy burdens, and I will give you rest. Take my yoke upon you. Let me teach you, because I am humble and gentle, and you will find rest for your souls. For my yoke fits perfectly, and the burden I give you is light'" (Matt. 11:28–30).

God never intended for you to push through your days and months feeling increasingly weary. If you are struggling with sleep disorders, there's hope! Let's take a look.

The benefits to your body and mind of plenty of restful sleep cannot be measured. Sleep is absolutely vital to your health and well-being. During sleep you actually recharge your mind and body. Sleep allows your body to recuperate and restore itself from exhaustion. In addition, during sleep your cells are able to regenerate, grow and rejuvenate because the body secretes growth hormones as you slumber that signal it to repair tissues and organs.

Sleep also gives your mind a mental break, and it helps to restore your memory. Dreaming helps your mind to sort out and resolve emotional conflicts. During sleep, your body rebuilds and removes toxins. As you rest your body mentally and physically, your energy is increased.

We spend up to one-third of our lives asleep, so getting adequate rest is critical for our health. Without enough sleep, the body begins to degenerate more rapidly. Adequate sleep actually helps to detoxify the brain by removing free radicals. If our brains are deprived of sleep over the long term, brain aging results.

Sleep deprivation and excessive fatigue can actually lead to anxiety, depression and extreme irritability, and can cause you to gain weight. Lack of sleep can also dramatically undermine your immune system, which leads to more colds, flus and other infectious diseases.

Fatigue will also lead to decreased mental functioning, causing problems at work or at school. The sleep-deprived tend to be more forgetful and less able to concentrate and focus. Decreased eye/hand coordination can result in a higher incidence of motor vehicle accidents. Tragically, about one hundred thousand accidents each year—resulting in nearly fifteen hundred deaths—are caused by people falling asleep at the wheel.

If you wake up never feeling rested and refreshed, you may be sleeping enough hours but still suffer from a sleep disorder that is robbing your body and mind of much-needed rest. Or if you drag through your days feeling tired and spend too many nights staring at the ceiling or wandering around your house, you may be one of millions of Americans who suffer from sleep disorders.

Sleep Disorders

Sleep disorders are at epidemic levels in the United States. An estimated sixty million Americans suffer from insomnia and other sleep disorders. Other reports state that more than half of all American adults suffer from insomnia at least a few times each week.[1] As a result, over 50 percent of the population will experience daytime drowsiness.

The average adult sleeps about seven to seven and a half hours a day during the work week. Sleep requirements vary from individual to individual. Some people are able to run on five hours of sleep a night, while others require nine or ten hours a night. The key is how you feel when you wake up and how alert you feel throughout your days. If you do not wake up feeling refreshed, and if you get sleepy during the day, you may be experiencing a sleep disorder.

A recent survey revealed that approximately one-third of all adults claimed they were so drowsy that it interfered with their daily activity activities. More than half of the American adult population experienced drowsiness during the day.[2]

These statistics may seem shocking, but sleep disorders don't have to happen to you! Many individuals live with insomnia, restless sleep, fatigue and mental cloudiness for years, believing that sleep disorders are something they must accept. But that is simply not true!

A Bold, New Approach

With the help of the practical and faith-inspiring wisdom contained in this Bible Cure booklet, you no longer have to suffer through sleepless nights or drag yourself through exhausted days. It's possible to start right now sleeping as soundly as a newborn baby—even if you've experienced sleep disorders for all of your life.

Through the power of good nutrition, healthy lifestyle choices, exercise, vitamins and supplements and, most importantly of all, through the power of dynamic faith, you can be empowered to sleep soundly and live in the robust health and vigor of a rested life.

Sleep disorders are not your destiny. With God's grace, energy, power and increasing joy await you!

As you read this book, prepare to win the battle against sleep disorders. This Bible Cure booklet is filled with practical steps, hope, encouragement and valuable information on how to develop a healthy, empowered lifestyle. In this book, you will

uncover God's divine plan of health
for body, soul and spirit
through modern medicine, good nutrition
and the medicinal power
of Scripture and prayer.

You will also discover life-changing scriptures throughout this booklet that will strengthen and encourage you.

As you read, apply and trust God's promises, you will also uncover powerful Bible Cure prayers to help you line up your thoughts and feelings with God's plan of divine health for you—a plan that includes living victoriously. In this Bible Cure booklet, you will find powerful insight in the following chapters:

1 Rest Assured—You Can Find Rest! 1
2 Rest Assured Through Nutrition 18
3 Rest Assured Through Exercise
   and Lifestyle Changes 30
4 Rest Assured Through Supplements . . .57
5 Rest Assured Through Rest in God 70

You can confidently take the natural and spiritual steps outlined in this book to combat and defeat sleep disorders forever.

It is my prayer that these practical suggestions for health, nutrition and fitness will bring wholeness to your life—body, soul and spirit. May they deepen your fellowship with God and strengthen your ability to worship and serve Him.

—Don Colbert, M.D.

A BIBLE CURE PRAYER
FOR YOU

Dear Lord, I give You all my sleepless nights and exhausted days. You said to come to You for rest, and as I enter the pages of this booklet, I ask You to help me to find rest in You. Help me to overcome fatigue and become energized to serve and worship You with my whole heart, mind, body and strength. Empower and strengthen me to find renewal in You for my body, mind and spirit. In Jesus' name, amen.

Chapter 1

Rest Assured—
You Can Find Rest!

Almighty God, who created the universe with unparalleled wisdom, also created your body to need rest. As a matter of fact, in His wisdom God made rest a foundational principle for life on earth. The Bible says, "On the seventh day, having finished his task, God rested from all his work. And God blessed the seventh day and declared it holy, because it was the day when he rested from his work of creation" (Gen. 2:2–3). Rest is a gift to all the earth's creatures to restore and refresh their physical and spiritual strength and to renew their vitality.

The rest your body needs is a vital part of living in God's divine health for you, and your loving Creator is committed to seeing that you get it. Take a moment and think about the heavenly Father's heart as you read these words: "The LORD is my shepherd, I shall not want. He makes me lie down in green pastures; He leads me beside quiet waters. He restores my soul" (Ps. 23:1–3, NAS).

If you are suffering because of not getting enough sleep, rest assured. God has provided wisdom to help you to gain a better

> *When thou liest down, thou shalt not be afraid: yea, thou shalt lie down, and thy sleep shall be sweet.*
> —PROVERBS 3:24, KJV

understanding of the reasons for your fatigue so that you can begin feeling much better very soon.

Understanding Sleep Deprivation

During my medical internship and residency I suffered tremendous sleep deprivation. I was on call all night long every third to fourth night. I often went through the night without sleeping, and then had to work the following day. During that season of my life I felt fatigued and drowsy much of the time.

Many professions in today's stressed-out world create fatigue and encourage sleep disorders. It is believed that a century ago the average person slept about eight or nine hours per night. Today, the average individual sleeps seven to seven and a half hours a night. Our modern lifestyles are so full that there's never enough time to get every-thing done, and consequently we tend to short ourselves on sleep. We end up paying for our many activities with drowsiness and fatigue.

Let's investigate how this gift from God, blessed sleep, really works and why it might not be working correctly for you.

Understanding How Sleep Works

To gain an understanding of sleep disorders it's critically important to understand the stages of sleep. Two main components of sleep exist. They are:

- Non–Rapid Eye Movement Sleep
- Rapid Eye Movement Sleep

As we investigate further, we'll just abbreviate Non–Rapid Eye Movement sleep as NREM and Rapid Eye Movement as REM for the sake of simplicity.

NREM

NREM is a cycle with four stages: stage one, stage two, stage three and stage four, with stage four being the deepest sleep. When you close your eyes and doze off, stage one begins.

REM

By the time you've entered stage five, you move into Rapid Eye Movement sleep. This is the level of sleep where dreaming takes place. During REM sleep the brain is very active. It is similar to being awake; in fact, the EEG brain waves are practically identical to being awake.

Completing a sleep cycle means that you've drifted from being in superficial stage one sleep all the way through stages two and three, and then you entered stage four, your deepest sleep. After that, you enter stage five, which is the dream stage. Each sleep cycle takes about ninety to a hundred minutes, and you usually complete about four or five sleep cycles during one night of sleep.

Cycling Through the Depths of Your Dreams

As you sleep your way through one cycle after another, the cycles change. More deep sleep (stages three and four) occurs in the first half of your sleep. Only a small amount of REM, or dream sleep, occurs. That means that the first half of your night is spent in deeper sleep.

As you gently slumber away, the length of REM sleep continues to increase and your sweet dreams last longer and longer as your brain works harder while dreaming. However, less and less time is spent in deep sleep (stages three and four) as daybreak approaches. When the little birds begin to chirp outside your window and light breaks forth, your dreaming sleep cycle of REM sleep can be lasting anywhere from thirty minutes to an hour.

Refreshing Dreams

Just as the dreams in your heart refresh your mind and energize your spirit during the day, your dreams at night refresh and restore as well.

However, the most restoring and recuperative stage of sleep occurs during the deeper stages of sleep—stages three and four. The other levels simply are your Cinderella's coach to take you there.

Stage one sleep is simply the drowsy stage in which you drift in and out of being awake. During stage one sleep it's easy to be awakened, for you are actually just dozing or are half-awake.

Stage two sleep, on the other hand, is a light level of sleep. Here your heart rate, respiratory rate and metabolic rate decrease. During stage two you can still be awakened easily.

Stage three sleep is the level where your breathing slows down. Your heart rate slows even more, and your muscles become more relaxed.

During this stage the body is able to regenerate, restore and repair organs and tissues due to the release of growth hormone.

You generally reach stage three sleep within thirty minutes of falling asleep. It's more difficult to awaken someone from stage three sleep. When you do wake them up, they tend to be a little groggy.

> *I will both lay me down in peace, and sleep: for thou, LORD, only makest me dwell in safety.*
> —PSALM 4:8, KJV

Stage four sleep is the deepest level of sleep, and it is the most restorative and refreshing form of sleep. This stage is reached approximately an hour after falling asleep, and it is by far the most important stage of sleep. After two to three sleep cycles, both stage three and stage four sleep may disappear for the remainder of the night. That's why it's critically important to get uninterrupted, peaceful, restorative sleep for the first three sleep cycles, which occur during the first four and a half hours of sleep. This is the best way to reap the benefit of this deep, restoring and repairing stage three and stage four sleep.

Sweet Dreams

The final stage is REM sleep, or dream sleep. During REM sleep the brain is much more active as the brain reacts to your dreams. In fact, the EEG tracing during REM sleep reveals rapid alpha waves, which are very similar to the brain waves that are present when you are awake. Your heart rate and respiratory rate may speed up a little during REM sleep.

A good night's sleep is just as important to your health as a healthy diet and regular exercise. But our modern lifestyles, often filled with worry, stress and many different pressures, can also lead to many types of sleep disorders. Insomnia is one of them.

What Sleep Disorder Do You Have?

Sleep disorders fall into two main categories:

- Dyssomnias
- Parasomnias

Dyssomnia

Dyssomnia is characterized by problems with either falling asleep or staying asleep followed by excessive drowsiness during the day. Examples of dyssomnias include insomnia, sleep apnea, narcolepsy, restless leg syndrome, periodic limb movements, hypersomnia and advanced and delayed sleep phase syndromes.

Parasomnias

Parasomnias, on the other hand, are simply abnormalities in behavior that occur during sleep such as grinding your teeth, night terrors (a frightening activity during sleep), sleepwalking and sleep talking.

Let's investigate some of these extremely unpleasant nighttime sleeping problems.

The Nightmare of Insomnia

As you start to doze off, a million different thoughts flood your head. The clock ticks more and more loudly as you wait to fall asleep. Hours seem to go by. Finally you get out of bed and get a drink or eat something, only to be confronted by the same sleeplessness when you return. By the time the sunlight breaks through the window, your eyes are burning, your brain is cloudy and you begin to panic over how you'll ever make it through the day at work feeling as you do. If you have ever suffered through nights such as these, chances are you're experiencing insomnia.

Insomnia sufferers may wake up an hour or two too early every morning or take an extra hour or two to fall asleep. It doesn't take long for insomnia to end up in sleep deprivation. If it continues, you'll find yourself exhausted in no time at all.

When You Cannot Fall Asleep

Insomnia is the most common sleep disorder. More than 50 percent of adults in the U.S. experience it at least a few times a week. If you are not able to fall asleep, or if you cannot stay asleep throughout the entire night, you probably have insomnia.

Insomnia can be further subdivided into three categories:

- Sleep-onset insomnia
- Sleep-maintenance insomnia
- Early-morning-awakening insomnia

This simply means that you have problems falling asleep and staying asleep, or you wake up too early in the morning and are unable to fall back to sleep. Insomnia can also be transient, which means it only occurs occasionally. It can be short term also, which is usually three nights to three weeks, or it can be chronic or long term.

Causes for Those Sleepless Nights

Insomnia has many different causes: medical causes such as chronic pain (especially arthritis), chronic back pain, fibromyalgia, degenerative disc disease and any other painful medical condition. Another common medical problem that commonly causes insomnia is benign prostatic hypertrophy, or simply an enlarged prostate.

Believe it or not, more than 80 percent of men between the ages of fifty and sixty have enlarged prostates. This condition causes such frequent trips to the bathroom at night that it commonly creates insomnia.

For women, menopause can be the culprit. Its trademark hot flashes in the middle of the night commonly cause insomnia. Women who suffer with painful menstrual cramping can experience bouts of insomnia as well.

Other health problems commonly associated with chronic sleeplessness include asthma, heart disease, respiratory disease, Alzheimer's disease and headaches.

Heartburn can be another culprit. Also called gastroesophageal reflux, heartburn is caused when stomach acids flow up into the esophagus during sleep. This can cause heartburn or a nighttime cough, which commonly causes insomnia.

Not all of insomnia's causes are physical. Psychological problems are a major factor. As much as 20 percent of the population will at some time be affected by anxiety or depression. Individuals suffering with anxiety often have difficulty getting to sleep and staying asleep. On the other hand, the depressed usually have trouble staying asleep. They usually wake up early, around 3 A.M., and have trouble falling back asleep. If you are experiencing either anxiety or depression, you can find more helpful information in my booklet *The Bible Cure for Depression and Anxiety*.

But I believe the most common cause of insomnia is excessive stress and tension. We will be discussing this in another chapter.

Mind Your Medications

Medications are also another common cause of insomnia. Here are some well-known culprits:

- Decongestants and other cold medications
- Appetite suppressants
- Certain antidepressants
- Theophylline
- Corticosteroids such as prednisone
- Amphetamines
- Estrogen-replacement drugs
- Thyroid hormones
- Some blood pressure medications
- Pain relievers containing caffeine, such as Excedrin

Is Dyssomnia Your Problem?

Let's briefly take a look at some other sleep disorders, called dyssomnias, that you may be battling.

Sleep apnea

Excessive snoring and brief moments when breathing stops completely are the telltale signs of this sleep disorder. Sleep apnea can wake you up several times during a night's sleep. Middle-aged men who are overweight are particularly prone to developing sleep apnea.

Although sleep apnea is associated with snoring, snoring alone does not indicate that you have it. Here are some other signs:

- Do you often find yourself falling asleep when you don't intend to, such as when you're driving or watching television?
- Have you had accidents because of sleepiness?
- Does excessive sleepiness interfere with your work or social life?
- Does your partner complain of your snoring and pauses in breathing at night?
- Do you awaken in the morning with a very dry mouth?

Periodic limb movement disorder

This disorder can wake you up several times throughout the night. It's characterized by either difficulty in falling asleep, excessive daytime sleepiness or even by falling asleep quickly but being restless all night. Sleeping partners may describe recurring movements of the legs or arms. These movements are usually an involuntary, repetitive jerking of the arms or legs that occurs suddenly while asleep.

- Have you been described as a restless sleeper?
- Do your arms or legs jerk frequently during sleep?
- Do you have trouble falling asleep?
- Does your partner tell you that you thrash around in your sleep?
- Are the sheets and bedcovers often disheveled or off your bed in the morning?

Narcolepsy

This relatively uncommon sleep disorder is quite serious. Narcolepsy is characterized by extreme daytime drowsiness and a tendency to fall asleep at inappropriate times. In addition, sufferers can experience a sudden loss of muscle strength or vivid dreams just before falling asleep or awakening. Double vision, memory loss and an inability to concentrate are other trademarks of this sleep disorder.

- Do you fall asleep during the day when you don't intend to?
- Do your muscles feel weak when you are excited, laughing or upset?
- Do you awaken from sleep with a feeling of paralysis?
- Do you see, hear or feel things when you are falling asleep or waking up?

If you suspect you could have narcolepsy, consult your physician.

Restless leg syndrome

This sleep disorder is sometimes described as discomfort in the calves and legs and a persistent urge to move the legs while sitting or lying in bed. Some say they feel a creepy, crawly sensation, a burning or other sensations. Some folks with restless leg syndrome also have periodic limb movement disorder, but those with periodic limb movement disorder often don't have restless leg syndrome.

- Do you feel the need to stretch or massage your legs?
- Do you have sensations while your legs are at rest and the feeling goes away with movement?
- Do you have trouble falling asleep with these feelings?

These are just a few of the more common sleep disorders. More than eighty different sleep disorders actually exist. If you experience any of these symptoms, do not be alarmed. Instead, choose to see it as the beginning point of your deliverance.

See Your Doctor

If you are experiencing a sleep disorder, it's important that you see your doctor. Get him or her to give you a thorough exam to rule out any serious medical or psychological problem that might be a factor.

Conclusion

Lying awake in the middle of the night trying to doze off can seem more miserable than nearly anything else. Still, your rest is very important to God, for it is a key principle of all that He created.

God desires that the earth and its creatures, whether great or small, enjoy blessed rest.

His wonderful Word says, "Work for six days, and rest on the seventh. This will give your ox and your donkey a chance to rest. It will also allow the people of your household, including your slaves and visitors, to be refreshed" (Exod. 23:12).

God promises to bless you with the gift of rest. With sound wisdom and God's help, I believe that you are beginning to put those endless nights of sleeplessness behind you!

A Bible Cure Prayer
FOR YOU

Dear Lord, I thank You that You have provided for my rest. If my way of living is breaking any of Your principles of health and sound wisdom, I ask You to help me to see it. Let my life line up in every way with Your perfect will so that I can enjoy the full benefits of Your blessed rest. Amen.

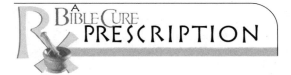

A BIBLE CURE PRESCRIPTION

Take this sleep habits quiz.[1] Circle the answer that best describes your week. The higher score the better. All 3s would indicate great sleep habits!

How much does your bedtime vary each night?
  1 Greatly
  2 Somewhat
  3 Very little

How much time are you spending awake in bed?
  1 A lot of time
  2 A little time
  3 Very little time

Are you napping too frequently and too long?
  1 Too many long naps
  2 Some naps
  3 Very few naps, if any

How consistent is your wake-up time?
  1 Very consistent
  2 Somewhat consistent
  3 Very inconsistent

How much are you hitting the snooze button?
  1 Way too much
  2 Every once in a while
  3 I don't use the snooze button

Are you waking up in the middle of the night for a reason (bathroom, hunger, going to bed too early)?
  1 Waking up too much
  2 Occasionally
  3 I rarely wake up

Chapter 2

Rest Assured Through Nutrition

Not only did God create the world to be founded upon a principle of rest, but He also created a dynamic display of delicious fruits, vegetables and many other foods to provide you with a wonderful array of nutritious choices. All that your body needs for divine health and rest has been bountifully provided for you by your loving heavenly Father. It's no wonder the psalmist declared, "Return to your rest, O my soul, for the LORD has dealt bountifully with you" (Ps. 116:7, NAS).

Learning how to use God's wisdom in giving your body the right nutritional selections can be a mighty key in breaking the power of sleep disorders and finding rest for your weary body and soul.

Let's take a look at how nutrition can help you.

Eating to Help Get Your Rest

What you eat and what you don't eat are major keys in how well you sleep, for nutrition and sleep are very much related.

Eating a healthy, well-balanced diet is vitally important for getting a good night's sleep. You should get plenty of B-complex vitamins, calcium, magnesium and other essential nutrients in your diet. Taking a comprehensive multivitamin such as Divine Health Multivitamin will enable you to obtain these nutrients.

In addition, if your diet is made up of fast foods and quick meals on the run, your body may not be getting enough L-tryptophan, which is a powerful amino acid that helps you sleep. Here's how it works. L-tryptophan is the amino acid that is the precursor to serotonin. Serotonin is a powerful chemical in your brain called a neurotransmitter that enables you to sleep. Tryptophan is also the precursor of melatonin, which also allows the body to sleep.

You can get L-tryptophan in yogurt, milk, meats (especially turkey), cashews, peanut butter, rice, bananas, whole-grain crackers, figs and dates.

Cut Caffeine

One of the most common causes of insomnia is

caffeine from coffee, tea, sodas or chocolate. Caffeine is a stimulant, and it actually increases the stress hormone epinephrine. This powerful substance can actually remain in the body up to twenty hours. More than 80 percent of all Americans consume caffeine regularly. The average American drinks about three cups of coffee per day.

Let's see how caffeine breaks down in some of the beverages you may be drinking regularly.

- Brewed coffee contains 110–130 milligrams of caffeine per 5 ounces.
- Tea contains about 60 milligrams of caffeine per 5 ounces.
- A 12-ounce Coke has about 65 milligrams of caffeine.
- A 12-ounce Mountain Dew has 52 milligrams of caffeine.
- A 12-ounce Jolt has 71 milligrams of caffeine.

Over-the-counter medications can be packed with caffeine as well. For example, one Excedrin contains 65 milligrams of caffeine. Cold medications also commonly contain caffeine.

Many people can drink caffeinated beverages without it affecting their sleep. However, just a little caffeine can cause severe insomnia in others. If you simply cannot get by without drinking caffeinated beverages, such as coffee, then be sure to drink them before noon. If you are battling insomnia and must have coffee, cut caffeine out of your diet except for one or two cups first thing in the morning shortly after awakening.

Too much caffeine can also predispose you to deficiencies in B vitamins, zinc, calcium, magnesium and iron. B vitamins calm the nerves and regulate L-tryptophan. Calcium and magnesium also help to relax the nervous system.

Alcohol and nicotine can also interfere with sleep. At first, alcohol may seem as if it helps a person to fall asleep. However, it later disrupts the stages of sleep by causing you to sleep lighter and wake up less refreshed.

Nicotine from cigarette smoking is a stimulant that causes adrenaline to be released into your system, causing insomnia.

Sleep Soundly With Less Sugar and Fewer Carbs

Caffeine is not the only dietary enemy of sleep. Sugar can be just as bad for your ability to rest. A poor diet of too many simple sugars and processed carbohydrates can also lead to insomnia. We in America eat far too much sugar, and when we eat sugar before going to bed, sleeplessness can be the result.

Americans are now consuming more fat-free foods, which usually means that they are

> *There remaineth therefore a rest for the people of God.*
> —HEBREWS 4:9, KJV

over-consuming highly processed carbohydrates and sugars. Foods high in processed carbohydrates and sugars stimulate insulin release from the pancreas. Insulin in turn triggers the body to store more fat. Insulin may also cause low blood sugar. Low blood sugar then triggers the adrenals to produce more adrenaline and cortisol, which may cause you to be awakened in the middle of the night.

Eating sugar and complex carbohydrates before bedtime often leads to low blood sugar in the middle of the night. This can also happen if you go to bed hungry. You can prevent this dip in blood sugar that wakes you out of sleep by eating a light, well-balanced snack at bedtime, such as a 40-30-30 supplement bar or a protein drink. Eating a light evening snack that is correctly balanced with proteins, carbohydrates and fats will stabilize blood sugar levels and improve sleep.

You may use whey protein, milk protein, soy or rice protein. Rice protein is the most hypoallergenic. There are protein powders that are correctly balanced 40 percent carbohydrate, 30 percent protein and 30 percent fat, such as Prozone, which may be mixed with water or skim milk. Or you may get plain protein powder such as whey, soy or rice (milk protein is more allergenic than the others) and make a smoothie.

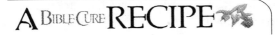

A BIBLE CURE RECIPE

DR. COLBERT'S PROTEIN SMOOTHIE

Here's a delicious protein smoothie that you can enjoy at bedtime. Not only will it help you to balance your blood sugar, but it will improve your health as well.

> 1–2 scoops protein powder, equal to 14–15 gr. protein
> ½ Tbsp. flaxseed oil or extra-virgin olive oil
> ½ frozen banana OR
>   1 cup frozen strawberries, raspberries, blackberries or blueberries
> ½ cup water or skim milk

Blend into a smoothie and enjoy!

Links Between Obesity and Insomnia

Many diseases are associated with insomnia, and these same diseases are closely related with obesity as well. Here's a list of these related diseases:

- Gastroesophageal reflux
- Heart disease
- Arthritis

Maintaining your ideal weight is another key to preventing these diseases, which in turn may prevent insomnia.

Maintaining Your Ideal Weight

Maintaining your ideal weight is critically important for sound sleep. More than 50 percent of American adults are either overweight or obese according to federal guidelines. Overweight is defined as a body mass index (BMI) of twenty-five to twenty-nine. Obesity is defined as a body mass index of thirty or more. The body mass index is simply a formula that considers your weight and height to determine if you are healthy, overweight or obese. Being overweight can definitely interfere with getting a good night's sleep.

You can find your own body mass index on the chart on page 25.

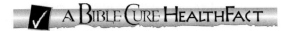

Body Mass Index

Too much body fat is an obvious warning sign. You can determine if you are overweight or obese with this body mass index (BMI) chart. Draw a line from your weight (left column) to your height (right column).

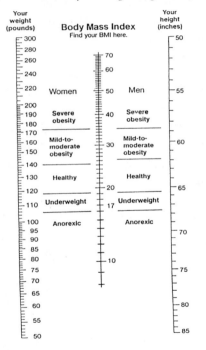

Your weight (pounds) — Body Mass Index — Find your BMI here. — Your height (inches)

Women / Men

Severe obesity

Mild-to-moderate obesity

Healthy

Underweight

Anorexic

Dinner Like a Pauper!

Never eat a large dinner just a few hours before bedtime. As your body labors to digest all that food, you can experience problems sleeping. It's best to eat breakfast like a king, lunch like a prince and dinner like a pauper. By eating a smaller dinner, your body is able to digest it faster. For more information on this balanced program, refer to my book *The Bible Cure for Weight Loss and Muscle Gain*.

When you choose your menu, be sure to keep in mind any food allergies that you may have. Food allergies or food sensitivities can create nighttime restlessness that leads to insomnia. The most common food allergies include milk, eggs, wheat products, yeast, chocolate, peanuts, corn and soy.

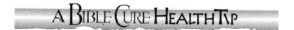

A BIBLE CURE HEALTH TIP

The Coca Pulse Test

Perform the Coca Pulse Test. Take your pulse for one minute prior to eating. Then place a bite of the food to which you might be allergic on your tongue. After thirty seconds, recheck your pulse. If the pulse rate goes up over six beats per minute you may be sensitive or allergic to the food. The higher the pulse goes up, usually the more severe the allergy or sensitivity.

Conclusion

One of the most powerful scriptures in the Bible is very short and simple. It says, "This I know, that God is for me" (Ps. 56:9, NAS). If ever you're tossing and turning at night or fighting the symptoms of a particular sleep disorder, let me encourage you to pull up this verse and never forget it. God is for you. He is on your side. He wants you to succeed in every way possible—in body, mind and spirit.

Before long you'll be declaring with the psalmist, "Return to your rest, O my soul, for the LORD has dealt bountifully with you" (Ps. 116:7, NAS).

> *At this, I woke up and looked around. My sleep had been very sweet.*
> —JEREMIAH 31:26

A Bible Cure Prayer
FOR YOU

*Dear Lord, thank You that You are with me
in everything that I do. Thank You for Your
care and concern in my life. Thank You for
Your great love and fatherly concern. Help
me to make all the changes I need to make
to my diet. And most of all, if ever I feel all
alone in the middle of the night, allow me
to feel Your presence to remind me that
You're always there. Amen.*

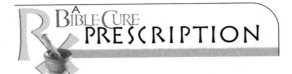

Describe your sleep disorder symptoms.

_____

_____

_____

What sleep disorder to do you feel that you are experiencing? (circle one)

Insomnia
Sleep apnea
Periodic limb movement disorder
Narcolepsy
Restless leg syndrome

Write a prayer thanking God that He is for you according to Psalm 116:7.

_____

_____

_____

_____

Chapter 3

Rest Assured Through Exercise and Lifestyle Changes

Every person and animal in God's creation must rest. The land and its plants rest as they cycle through seasons. As a foundational principle of creation, God designed rest to strengthen every aspect of your life and health. The Bible says, "For thus the Lord GOD, the Holy One of Israel, has said, 'In repentance and rest you shall be saved, in quietness and trust is your strength'" (Isa. 30:15, NAS).

Getting the rest you need is vital to everything you do. Rest heals and restores your body, and rest in God saves or delivers you from the pressures and stress that daily assault your spirit and mind.

Dealing with that stress and pressure through exercise and a number of valuable lifestyle changes may be all that you need to once again enjoy the refreshing rest you need. Let's turn and look at the connection between your lifestyle and rest.

Are You Losing Sleep Over Stress?

Probably one of the most common causes of insomnia is an excessive amount of stress. We live in such a fast-paced society. We have less and less time to complete more and more tasks. Like the ancient Israelites under the harsh rule of Pharaoh, our stressed-out American lifestyle seems to be constantly demanding that we produce more and more bricks with less and less straw.

This leaves most Americans under constant stress. There is stress in the home, such as teenagers, marital conflict, financial pressures and family conflict. There is stress at the job with deadlines, quotas and competition. There is traffic stress and financial stress. Also, having a child with ADD, a child on drugs or a child with problems in school will add extra stress. Combine normal, everyday stress with unexpected emotional stress such as an

> *I urge you therefore, brethren, by the mercies of God, to present your bodies a living and holy sacrifice, acceptable to God, which is your spiritual service of worship.*
> —ROMANS 12:1, NAS

unexpected illness, accident, divorce or separation, serious illness in the family, loss of job, a lawsuit or any other major financial stress, and life can get pretty overwhelming.

Far too often stress leaves us staring at the ceiling in the dark trying to get our sleep. Much of modern life is a recipe for insomnia. About 70 or 80 percent of patient visits to doctors' offices are for stress-related problems.[1]

Understanding Stress

Many people respond to excess stress by overeating, smoking, drinking alcohol, becoming depressed and anxious or by losing sleep. But not all stress is bad. As a matter of fact, some stress is very good, and the right amount of stress is healthy.

Think of stress as similar to tuning the strings of a guitar. If the strings are too tight, they will break. If they are too loose, the instrument will not make good music. If you are competing in a basketball, softball or golf tournament, or any other type of sport, the right amount of stress will actually help you to perform better.

Your Body and the Stages of Stress

The body responds to stress by the general adaptation syndrome. This was actually described in 1956 by Dr. Hans Selye in the book *The Stress of Life.*[2] In the general adaptation syndrome there are three stages.

The alarm stage

The alarm stage is characterized by the fight-or-flight response. During the alarm stage, the autonomic nervous system and the endocrine system become stimulated.

The autonomic nervous system consists of two branches: the sympathetic nervous system and the parasympathetic nervous system. The sympathetic nervous system is stimulated during the alarm stage.

When your sympathetic nervous system becomes excited, your heart rate increases and you begin breathing faster. Your mind becomes very alert and your blood pressure rises. Blood sugars increase to supply fuel for the muscles, getting them ready for fight or flight. Perspiration increases and digestive secretions decrease.

During the alarm stage hormones flood into your bloodstream—especially adrenaline and cortisol.

Adrenaline raises blood pressure and increases heart rate, respiratory rate and metabolic rate. In this way, adrenaline provides extra energy and strength to either fight or flee. The hormone cortisol is also stimulated.

Nevertheless, the alarm stage is usually very brief. When you feel safe again from the perceived danger you settle back down, and all the body systems relax back to their former peaceful state.

Historically, this alarm reaction served us well. We were able to fight off attackers or run from trouble. But modern-day Americans can undergo these same reactions on a daily basis as they drive in traffic or go through their stressful daily routines.

These high-energy hormones are continually being stimulated throughout the day for low-energy needs. In other words, you are continually wasting a dollar's worth of energy for a two-cent problem.

For instance, if you were to see a six-foot rattlesnake coming toward you as you walked out to your car in the parking lot, this alarm reaction would go off and you would turn and run. Likewise, if you were camping and encountered a bear, this alarm reaction would, again, go off and could save your life by enabling you to run to safety. However, minor problems such as an argument with your spouse or teenage son, a driver cutting you off in traffic or a back-stabbing fellow employee at work can stimulate the same alarm reaction throughout the day, resulting in increased stress and increased fatigue.

Resistance stage

If these alarm reactions continue to occur frequently throughout the day, you may eventually feel that you have little or no control and give up. At this point, you have reached the stage of stress called the resistance stage.

An example of this is an employee who has no hope for promotion. He hates his job but continues to work to pay his bills. He perceives that he has lost control and has no way out. Perhaps a family can be so far into debt that they have given up and have lost all hope of getting out of debt. You can see that many individuals who are experiencing high degrees of stress end up with negative, failure mentalities that cause them to give up.

This perceived loss of control over a long period of time stimulates the sympathetic nervous system. It also continually stimulates the adrenal glands, which causes a prolonged increase of both cortisol and adrenaline. This leads to prolonged elevation of both cortisol and adrenaline levels in the body. Under normal conditions, cortisol is secreted in daily cycles. It usually peaks in the morning and is at its lowest levels at night.

The Dangers of Too Much Cortisol

High levels of cortisol are closely related to insomnia and sleep disorders. Elevated cortisol levels also lead to elevated blood sugar, increased bone loss, increased accumulation of fat around the waist, decreased muscle tone, an elevation in triglycerides and cholesterol, impaired immune function and a greater susceptibility to allergies.

Is Your Insomnia Stress Related?

Researchers have found that about 41 percent of all insomnia is linked to stress or other emotional factors.[3] Over the long run, having too much cortisol and adrenaline in your bloodstream eventually depletes the supply. Sooner or later your adrenal glands will become exhausted as cortisol and adrenaline levels decrease due to the inability of the adrenal glands to keep up with the high demand of producing these powerful hormones. When this happens, you begin to enter into the third stage of stress.

Adrenal exhaustion stage

A prolonged decrease of both adrenaline and cortisol leads to insomnia and awakening in the middle of the night. This is the most dangerous stage of the general adaptation syndrome. If you remain in this stage too long, you may eventually experience extreme fatigue, irritability, immune dysfunction and low blood sugar. At this point your body begins to break down, resulting in recurrent infections, worsening of allergies, autoimmune diseases (such as lupus, rheumatoid arthritis and MS) and even cancer.

If you are experiencing insomnia due to stress, it's critically important to identify which stage of stress you are in. Is it the alarm stage, the resistance stage or the exhaustion stage? Your doctor can help you to determine this through tests designed especially for this purpose.

Stress Busters

When you realize what stress does to your body, it's certainly not difficult to understand how important it is to deal with your stress, especially if it's so severe that it's keeping you up at night. Here are some stress-busting ideas that can help.

Deep-breathing exercises

You can dramatically reduce your stress by taking just a few minutes every day to perform some deep-breathing exercise. Simply lie down on your bed with your eyes closed and concentrate on your breathing. Place a book on your abdomen in order to properly perform abdominal breathing relaxation exercises.

- Inhale slowly through the nose over four seconds.
- Expand the muscles of the abdomen first. (The book should rise in the air.)
- Expand your chest with air.
- Hold your breath for about four seconds.
- Slowly exhale through the mouth and feel the chest and abdomen contract. (The book should sink as the air is exhaled.)

All deep-breathing exercises should be belly breathing or diaphragmatic breathing. Belly breathing or diaphragmatic breathing uses the diaphragm and abdominal muscles instead of the chest muscles. With practice, you can inhale for ten, twenty and even thirty seconds.

Progressive relaxation

Another great stress-buster is a progressive relaxation technique that was developed by Dr. Jacobsen.[4] You can perform this exercise anywhere—sitting at your desk, lying on your bed or reclining on your couch.

- Contract one group of muscles for a few seconds and then relax them.
- Take a deep breath as you tighten the muscles.
- Relax as you exhale.

It is best to begin with the toes and work up to the calves, the thighs, abdomen, chest, arms, shoulders, neck and face. Focus your attention on contracting your muscles for a few seconds and then relaxing them; don't allow your mind to wander, but focus on your breathing and also on flexing and relaxing your muscles. Your stress will melt away.

Aerobic exercise

Aerobic exercise such as brisk walking is one of the best ways to improve the quality of your sleep. Aerobic exercise helps you to fall asleep faster and to sleep longer. Those who exercise regularly also spend a greater amount of time in stage three and stage four sleep, which are the most restorative, repairing stages of sleep.

> *Six days you are to do your work, but on the seventh day you shall cease from labor in order that your ox and your donkey may rest, and the son of your female slave, as well as your stranger, may refresh themselves.*
> —Exodus 23:12, NAS

By spending more time in stages three and four sleep you will awaken more refreshed and have much more energy throughout the day. However, don't exercise within three hours of bedtime for this can actually cause insomnia.

You don't have to join a gym. Simply take a brisk walk, cycle, go dancing or get involved in any other aerobic activity that elevates the heart rate for about twenty to thirty minutes four times a week. This will help you to lose weight, reduce stress and improve your sleep.

Choose an aerobic exercise that you enjoy, and you won't become bored with it. Get a partner—a friend or your spouse—and if you choose walking, vary your experiences by going to different parks or malls for a change of scenery. Walk slowly enough so that you can carry on a conversation, but quickly enough so that you cannot sing. Over time, you should notice that your sleep improves dramatically.

Learn to calculate your training heart rate. Once you have determined your desired heart rate range, write down your actual heart rate after each aerobic session.

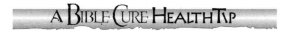

A BIBLE CURE HEALTH TIP

Your Predicted Heart Rate

Calculate your predicted heart rate using this formula:

220 minus [your age] = _____

x .65 = _____ x .80 = _____

Calculate your target heart zone using this formula:

220 minus [your age] = _____

x .65 = _____

[This is your minimum.]

220 minus [your age] = _____

x .80 = _____

[This is your maximum.]

This example may help: To calculate the target heart zone for a 40-year-old man, subtract the age (40) from 220 (220- 40=180). Multiply 180 by .65, which equals 117. Then multiply 180 by .80, which equals 144. A 40-year-old man's target heart rate zone is 117–144 beats per minute.

Planning Your Sleep Environment

In addition to getting exercise, making some changes to your sleep environment will also help you to sleep better.

Limit your bedroom to sleep.

For starters, begin using your bedroom for sleep only. Don't study, eat, work on a computer, watch television or do any other activity in your bedroom but sleep. When you go to bed and happen to look at your computer or fax machine before you doze off, you may actually feel stressed by thinking of the work that you need to do, and this can lead to insomnia.

Most patients claim that watching TV does not cause insomnia, but there is always a percentage of patients with insomnia aggravated by watching TV in the bedroom. These patients definitely sleep better without a TV in the bedroom. Patients with insomnia should also avoid action-packed movies, thrillers or sports before bedtime since they get the adrenaline flowing.

Keep your bedroom uncluttered.

In addition, try to keep your bedroom uncluttered as much as possible to avoid distractions that may cause stress.

Only read if it helps you to sleep.

Reading the Bible or a novel may also help you to fall asleep. For others, reading can keep them up. Therefore, only read if it helps you to fall asleep.

Don't go to bed unless you are sleepy.

If you're not sleepy when bedtime comes, do some relaxing activity until you get sleepy. Try taking a warm bath, reading the Bible, having a massage, performing simple stretching exercises or any other activity that helps you to wind down.

Keep your bedroom dark.

A dark bedroom is essential in creating the

right atmosphere for sleep. Make sure that your bedroom is very dark with no light shining into it from the street or from even a nightlight. You may even need to cover your digital clock since clocks are usually lighted. Be sure that your drapes or curtains are lined or that you have a dark shade to pull to block any light from a streetlight or car headlights.

Remove noise.

Your sleep should be free of distracting noises, ringing phones, honking horns, sirens and other sounds that could disrupt your sleep. Remember, if your sleep is interrupted during the deeper stages of sleep, you may lose the benefits of that sleep cycle or you may not be able to fall back to sleep.

If you cannot control some of the noise, get a machine that reproduces sounds such as the ocean waves, waterfall or raindrops, or even white noise. Or you can purchase a Hepa Air Filter that produces a gentle humming noise that drowns out background noise.

If the telephone is a problem, take it off the hook when you retire.

Is the temperature cozy?

Keep your bedroom at a comfortable temperature, which is usually around seventy degrees.

Many people prefer a ceiling fan to improve airflow. However, the key is that you should feel comfortable—neither too hot, nor too cold, nor too humid. If your feet get cold, make sure you wear warm socks.

Get rid of the Goldilocks complex.

Is your bed too hard, soft, big or little? Be sure that your bed is comfortable for both you and your spouse to sleep on. Is the mattress firm enough to support your body weight? It should support your lower back and keep your spine in alignment. Also, make sure that it's cushiony enough to allow you to sleep soundly.

Remember, you are going to spend approximately one-third of your life in bed. Make sure that your mattress and pillow are the most comfortable ones that you can afford. One of the best investments in your health is a very good mattress that enables you to sleep comfortably.

What about your pillow?

Is your pillow too small, hard, soft or large for your comfort? Carefully select a pillow that's right for you. Make sure it's not overstuffed and that it's able to support both your head and neck, keeping them in alignment with the spine.

By performing these simple measures of

creating the right atmosphere for sleep, many cases of insomnia are cleared up.

Does Your Partner's Snoring Keep You Awake?

Does your partner happily saw logs all night while you watch the ceiling? If your spouse snores, it could be sign of sleep apnea. Have your partner undergo a medical evaluation if he or she seems to stop breathing for short periods of time.

Snoring that is not related to sleep apnea does not pose any health risks and does not cause daytime drowsiness for the snorer. However, it does for the snorer's spouse. Snoring is also fairly difficult to cure.

Snoring is one of the most common sleep problems in the U.S., affecting about 25 percent of men and 12 percent of women. Those who snore often have anatomical differences such as an obstructed nasal passage or an elongation of the uvula (which is the tissue that hangs down the back of the throat), or it may be due to sagging of the soft palate. Enlarged tonsils or

> *Indeed, he who watches over Israel never tires and never sleeps.*
> —Psalm 121:4

45

adenoids can cause snoring also, as well as poor muscle tone in the tissues of the soft palate, throat and tongue.

Changing sleeping positions can help. Try sewing a pocket into the back of a T-shirt and placing a tennis ball in it to keep your happy snorer from sleeping on his back.

Since most snorers tend to be overweight and have increased girth of the neck and poor muscle tone of the tongue and throat, losing weight and exercising is the best advice for snorers—a weight loss of just ten to fifteen pounds can make a big difference! Avoid alcohol, muscle relaxants, tranquilizers and sleep medications since they tend to relax the muscles of the throat, which can worsen snoring. Many snorers have nasal congestion, and Breathe Rite strips, a decongestant or a nasal steroid such as Flonase or Nasonex will help to open the nasal passages and may prevent snoring. Cigarette smoke can also cause the tissues of the throat to swell and thus encourage snoring.

If none of these ideas work, try a dental appliance, which helps about 60 percent of the snorers. Or, you can also purchase a snore alarm at Shaper Image. A snore alarm is simply a wristwatch that vibrates as soon a person begins to snore.

For a non-snoring spouse try a background noise machine (which can also be purchased at Sharper Image). With it the noise of a waterfall, raindrops or white noise can drown out a snoring spouse. You might also get some soft earplugs until your snoring partner has been treated.

Obstructive Sleep Apnea

Even though all patients with sleep apnea snore, all snorers do not have sleep apnea. Obstructive sleep apnea is the most common type of this very serious disorder, occurring in about 2 to 4 percent of all middle-aged adults. More than 80 percent of those with sleep apnea don't even realize they suffer from it!

In this condition the upper airway becomes completely obstructed for ten seconds or longer. It may happen a few times each night, or it can occur hundreds of times. During these episodes, blood levels of oxygen decrease and carbon dioxide levels increase.

> *The sleep of the working man is pleasant, whether he eats little or much. But the full stomach of the rich man does not allow him to sleep.*
> —ECCLESIASTES 5:12, NAS

It's this change in the blood gases that alerts the

sleeper's brain to start breathing again. But for this to occur the brain must awaken the body from sleep. These apneic episodes may occur twenty to hundreds of times a night, awaking the sleeper each time—although he may not realize it. As you can imagine, the result is daytime drowsiness, depression and learning and memory problems. It's also linked to irregular heartbeats, high blood pressure, heart attacks and strokes.

About 60 percent or more of those with sleep apnea are seriously overweight. In addition, if a man or woman has a large neck, a double chin and truncal obesity (obesity around the abdominal region), there seems to be an increased correlation with obstructive sleep apnea also. The larger the neck size and the more alcohol that is consumed, the higher the correlation with this sleep disorder.

The most common treatment for sleep apnea is a CPAP machine with a face mask. However, about 50 percent of patients with obstructive sleep apnea benefit from laser surgery (and even newer techniques) to decrease the size of the uvula, soft palate or both. But the most important treatment for sleep apnea is losing weight and avoiding alcohol, tranquilizers, muscle relaxants and sleep aids. If you suspect that you or your spouse has sleep apnea, consult your doctor and have a sleep study performed.

As you lose weight, be sure that you exercise to decrease your neck size. Additional information on this subject can be found in my booklet *The Bible Cure for Weight Loss and Muscle Gain*.

Light Up Your Life!

The body's clock is actually located in a part of the brain called the hypothalamus. Sunlight plays a very important part in influencing your body's clock rhythms, called circadian rhythms. Alarm clocks and artificial light sources such as full spectrum lights can be used to set your body clock and influence your circadian rhythms.

Circadian rhythms are also influenced by the time we choose to go to bed, the time we choose to wake up, the timing of our meals and the timing of our exercise and of our nightlife.

Circadian rhythms are influenced by many factors that vary from person to person. That's why some of us are early birds and others are night owls. Early birds are more alert and active during the day, especially in the morning. They usually begin to settle down in the evening. Early birds usually enjoy breakfast and are much sharper mentally in the morning hours.

The night owls, on the other hand, stay up into the wee hours of the morning and then sleep late. These folks often skip breakfast and rely on coffee to get them going. They usually perform poorly in the morning and become mentally alert and more energetic in the afternoon.

Night owls should choose jobs that allow them to work in the afternoon and evening hours. Or they can attempt to change their time clocks and their circadian rhythms by going to bed earlier, waking up earlier, using light therapy, improving their diet, decreasing their stress and starting a regular exercise program.

Light Therapy
for Improving Sleep

Believe it or not, how much bright sunlight you get during the day can have a significant impact on how well you sleep!

Most Americans spend way too much time indoors with dim artificial light or florescent lighting. Consequently, we get far too little bright sunlight. This disrupts our circadian clocks, which alters our mood, interferes with our sleep and affects us both mentally and physically.

Low amounts of natural light exposure for a prolonged period of time will eventually cause an imbalance of the hormones serotonin and melatonin. This can lead to Seasonal Affective Disorder, otherwise known as SAD. SAD involves experiencing a mild depression with symptoms of sadness, hopelessness, lethargy, weight loss or weight gain and other symptoms of mild depression.

Those with SAD really are sad. This disorder usually occurs during autumn and winter months when days grow shorter, thus limiting sunlight.

Also called winter depression, SAD affects about ten million Americans each year. These people need more sleep; they experience a decreased quality of sleep and wake up tired. Seasonal Affective Disorder is much more common in the northern part of the U.S.

Getting enough sunlight during the day will help increase melatonin at night. It also helps to

> *Casting all your care upon Him, for He cares for you.*
> —1 PETER 5:7, NKJV

increase the neurotransmitters serotonin and norepinephrine. Melatonin and serotonin help to promote sleep, whereas norepinephrine and serotonin also help to elevate your mood.

51

Spend at least thirty minutes to one hour a day in the sunlight. You can eat lunch outside at a picnic table or inside near a window that allows plenty of sunlight in. If you live in the North where many days are overcast, it might help to purchase a light box that has full spectrum lights. If you live in sunny southern climates where adequate sunlight is abundant, then sit outside at lunch for approximately thirty minutes to an hour under a shade tree and receive the healing power of light as you enjoy your lunch.[5]

Night-shift workers

If you work evenings, night shifts or rotating shifts, a few changes may help—especially if you work rotating shifts. If you work at night and sleep during the day, be sure to sleep in a completely dark room with all light sealed out. Before you leave for work in the evening, spend time in a light box, or spend time wearing a light visor. Finally, when you return home in the morning, wear dark sunglasses to prepare the mind and body for sleep.

For those who tend to work crazy hours, napping can be a godsend. Let's look. Also, an excellent program for insomnia is Good Night America. For more information about this program, call 1-877-211-REST.

Power Napping

During my last year of high school I lived in Mexico as an exchange student. Every afternoon after lunch we would take a siesta or nap for about an hour and a half. Many people get drowsy in the midafternoon, and taking a nap can help refresh and rejuvenate their minds as well as their bodies.

This fact is catching on in the business world. Some companies now have napping facilities. This is usually a room that is dark, free of distractions and filled with comfortable recliners or cots.

Since so many Americans are sleep deprived, napping is one of the best ways for restoring and catching up on sleep.

However, only take a nap if you feel drowsy. Either take a very short nap, which is usually less than thirty minutes, or a long nap, which is usually around ninety minutes.

A 30-wink power nap

You can get refreshed and restored by napping for just about a half-hour. A nap of less than thirty minutes allows your body to go through stages one and two of the sleep cycle. If you sleep beyond that and wake up in stages three and four or REM sleep, you probably will feel pretty groggy or more fatigued for the rest of the day.

A siesta

If you take a nap for ninety minutes, your body can go through all stages of sleep and complete an entire sleep cycle. This leaves you feeling more

> *Give heed to me, and answer me; I am restless in my complaint and am surely distracted.*
> —PSALM 55:2, NAS

refreshed and rejuvenated. Use a watch alarm or set your pager on vibration mode to help you wake up from your power nap.

Tips for Power Nappers

When power napping, it's extremely important to deal with all possible distractions. Unplug phones. Get the room as dark as possible, and get in a comfortable position on a couch or recliner.

Done correctly, a power nap can leave you feeling refreshed and regenerated mentally and recharged physically for the remainder of the day. But never take a power nap too late in the day, or it will interfere with your sleep at night. Early afternoon or midafternoon is the best time for napping.

Conclusion

By now you've discovered that many of your daily choices can impact your ability to walk in the wonderful blessing of refreshing, rejuvenating sleep. Enjoying rest is a powerful gift from God. Therefore, always look to Him for blessed rest, for He promises to give you sleep. The Bible says, "It is vain for you to rise up early, to sit up late, to eat the bread of sorrows; for so He gives His beloved sleep" (Ps. 127:2, NKJV).

A BIBLE CURE PRAYER FOR YOU

I thank You, God, that You promised me blessed, quiet, refreshing and rejuvenating rest because You love me. Show me what lifestyle changes I need to make to walk in the blessings of Your gift of rest. Help me to develop a regular exercise routine, and help me to stick to it once I've begun. I thank You with all my heart for Your great and mighty love for me. Help me to order my life in a way that always pleases You. Amen.

R BIBLE CURE PRESCRIPTION

Here are ten tremendous tips you can take to help you sleep.[6] Check the ones you plan to use.

- ❏ Stay away from the big four: caffeine, stress, alcohol and smoking.
- ❏ Leave time in your schedule for sleep.
- ❏ Set a regular sleep schedule, seven days a week. Get up at the same time every day.
- ❏ Relax before going to bed. Reflect on the day, release your stress and plan for tomorrow.
- ❏ Use your bedroom for sleep only—no work, study or eating. If the TV causes insomnia, get it out of the bedroom.
- ❏ Prepare a comfortable sleep environment with a comfortable pillow, mattress and room temperature. Remove all noise and light from the bedroom.
- ❏ Start a regular exercise program, but don't exercise for three to four hours before bedtime.
- ❏ Observe good eating habits. Don't go to bed hungry, and don't drink excessive fluids before bed.
- ❏ Get up if you can't sleep after twenty to thirty minutes and go to another room to relax. Return to bed when you are tired.
- ❏ Determine to make sleep a priority and regular part of your life.

Chapter 4

Rest Assured Through Supplements

God promises sweet sleep to those who conduct their lives with His wisdom. The Bible says, "Keep sound wisdom and discretion, so they will be life to your soul, and adornment to your neck . . . When you lie down, you will not be afraid; when you lie down, your sleep will be sweet" (Prov. 3:21–22, 24, NAS).

One way to walk in wisdom is to understand good stewardship of your own health by providing your body with all it needs for proper sleep. In addition, learn what nutrients, herbs and other supplements can help.

Supplementing your diet with vitamins, minerals, herbs and other supplements can dramatically impact many sleep disorders. So let's take a look at a program of supplementation that will make you wiser about helping your body to sleep.

Supplements for Sound Sleep

To begin a supplementation program, be sure that your body has all the vitamins and minerals it needs to function at optimal levels. Start with a good overall multivitamin/multimineral supplement.

A good multivitamin/multimineral supplement

I strongly recommend a comprehensive multivitamin and multimineral supplement that contains adequate levels of B vitamins, magnesium, calcium and trace minerals. Usually a vitamin containing 50 milligrams of each B vitamin, 400 milligrams of magnesium, 800 milligrams of calcium, 30 milligrams of zinc and 2–3 milligrams of copper, in addition to the other essential vitamins and minerals, will provide optimal nutritional supplementation for a good night's sleep. Divine Health Multivitamin for men and women is an excellent multivitamin.

Several special herbs and other supplements are especially effective in helping you sleep. However, never become completely dependent upon any supplement in order to sleep. Use supplements until you find and correct the cause for your sleep disorder, and then discontinue using the supplements. Let's look at some of these helpful supplements.

Valerian

Valerian is an herb that has been used for centuries in Europe for sleep. Several studies have demonstrated that valerian is able to relieve insomnia and improve the quality of sleep.[1] However, valerian keeps a very small percentage of people awake. Therefore, if you find it seems to stimulate you instead of helping you sleep, stop using it right away.

Take 150–400 milligrams of valerian about an hour before bedtime.

Passionflower

Passionflower is an herb that is commonly taken with valerian. Passionflower helps to relieve anxiety and also has sedative effects.

Take 300–450 milligrams an hour before bedtime.

Hops

Hops is the source of beer's bitterness, but it also has been used to treat insomnia. Hops is normally combined with passionflower or valerian since it only has a mild sedative effect.

Take 500–1000 milligrams an hour prior to

bedtime, or you may drink hops tea, which is available from a health food store.

Kava

Kava is an herb that has antianxiety and sedative effects. Several double-blind studies have shown that kava helps to improve anxiety.[2] Since anxiety is a common cause of insomnia, I may place patients with insomnia due to anxiety on kava.

Take 210 milligrams an hour prior to bedtime. Or you may take 70–100 milligrams of kava three times a day. (The kava extract needs to be standardized to 70 percent kavalactones, which is the active ingredient.)

St. John's wort

St. John's wort has been used in Europe for a number of years to treat depression. In fact, in Germany it is commonly prescribed for depression. St. John's wort is also used in the treatment of chronic insomnia when it's related to depression. St. John's wort is able to maintain serotonin levels in the brain. Purchase a variety containing 0.3 percent hypericin, which is usually quite effective in relieving insomnia caused by depression. However, it usually takes four weeks before the full effect is realized.

Take 300 milligrams, three times a day. Although side effects are quite rare, if you experience any, simply stop taking this herb. Do not take St. John's wort with any other antidepressant medications, such as Prozac, Zoloft and Paxil.

5-HTP

5-HTP increases the time you spend in the deep, refreshing stages three and four of your sleep. It also increases REM sleep. 5-HTP is also used to treat depression since it raises levels of serotonin.

You may take 100–300 milligrams of 5-HTP one hour before retiring. Always start with the lowest dose and gradually increase it to promote and maintain sleep. Please do not take 5-HTP if you are taking any other antidepressant medication.

Getting Into Rhythm!

Whether you know it or not, you have rhythm! Each of us has our own slightly different internal biological clock controlling our circadian rhythms. These are simply rhythms that occur regularly— about every twenty-four hours. As we saw earlier, circadian rhythms are associated with biological changes in our bodies such as fluctuations in temperature, hormonal levels and a raft of other biological changes that impact the way we feel throughout the day.

An example of hormonal fluctuations due to circadian rhythms is the way melatonin is secreted by the pineal gland in the brain. Melatonin usually reaches its peak around 2 A.M., and then it begins to drop off around 4 A.M.

Your melatonin supply also fluctuates throughout your lifetime. Melatonin levels are higher during childhood and usually peak

> *The steadfast of mind Thou wilt keep in perfect peace.*
> —ISAIAH 26:3, NAS

at about age ten, which is closely related to growth spurts that are commonly associated with an increased need of sleep. During adolescence, melatonin levels start to decline, and this decline continues for the rest of your life. People over sixty produce very low amounts of melatonin and usually need supplementation. I commonly place individuals over sixty years of age on melatonin, 1–3 milligrams sublingual, at bedtime.

Many other hormones undergo circadian rhythms. For example, the stress hormone cortisol, which is produced by the adrenal gland, begins to rise in the early morning usually as melatonin levels start to fall. As cortisol rises, you wake up.

People with normal circadian rhythms are alert mainly in the morning and afternoon. They tend to get sleepy in the evening due to the body's biological changes over twenty-four hours.

Melatonin

Many people say that melatonin supplements really help them to fall asleep and stay asleep, but others insist that melatonin has absolutely no effect on them. The fact is that if your own body's melatonin levels are low, this supplement may really help you to sleep. However, if you already have plenty of melatonin, it will probably have little effect.

Melatonin can really help those who suffer with jet lag, night shift workers and others who struggle with sleep when their lives demand that they reset their biological clocks.

However, melatonin causes unpleasant side effects in some folks, including nightmares, agitation, anxiety, drowsiness or grogginess the next day. If any of these symptoms occur, stop using melatonin immediately.

A dose of 1–3 milligrams at bedtime is usually adequate.

Getting Started
With Sleep Supplements

Again, I want to emphasize that herbs and supplementation should be used on a short-term basis unless you have anxiety or depression, or if you are over the age of sixty and are deficient in melatonin. This is how I suggest using supplements to help you get beyond the present fatigue of sleep disorders.

- I initially start patients with insomnia on 5-HTP, 100–300 milligrams approximately an hour before bedtime.

- I may then add valerian and passionflower, approximately an hour before bedtime if the insomnia persists.

- For elderly people, I start with melatonin, 1–3 milligrams sublingual, at bedtime.

- If you have insomnia and depression, take 300 milligrams of St. John's wort three times a day.

- If you are experiencing anxiety or excessive stress, take kava.

Supplements for Other Sleep Disorders

Since so many sleep disorders exist, let's look beyond insomnia to some of the less-common sleep disorders. Although these other disorders can seem very frustrating and impossible to change, supplements can help a lot.

Restless leg syndrome

If you are experiencing restless leg syndrome, get your doctor to test you to see if your body is low in iron. A test called a ferritin level blood test can measure the iron stores in your body. If your ferritin level is low, supplementing iron may relieve restless leg syndrome. Regular aerobic exercise, leg massages and warm baths with Epsom salts can also help relieve the symptoms of restless leg syndrome.

Periodic limb movement disorder

Periodic limb movement disorder commonly occurs with restless leg syndrome. This involuntary disorder often causes repetitive, jerking twitches of the legs that last between one and three seconds. This twitching can wake up the sleeper or his or her spouse. Those with this disorder tend to feel quite drowsy throughout the day.

Here are some supplements that can help:

- Take 400 milligrams of magnesium in the form of magnesium citrate, magnesium aspartate or magnesium glycinate at bedtime.

- Take 800 units of vitamin E daily.

In addition, taking a warm bath and adding 2–4 cups of Epsom salts to the bath water can also help.

Should I Ask My Doctor
for Medications for Sleep?

I do not routinely recommend pharmaceutical medications for insomnia since they often have side effects. These include addiction or dependence upon the drug, rebound insomnia and disrupting the normal architecture of sleep.

Rebound insomnia occurs when the insomnia becomes even worse after you go off the medication. Disrupting sleep architecture means that some sleep medications will make you fall asleep, but you will not spend adequate time in the deeper stages, such as stages three and four. Instead, most of your sleep time will be spent in the superficial stages, such as stages one and two.

However, newer medications, including Ambien

and Sonata, have fewer side effects and are very beneficial for treating insomnia on a short-term basis.

Conclusion

The promise of living wisely includes enjoying the benefits of refreshing, restoring sweet sleep. Dragging through your days fatigued and tossing through your nights awake is not healthy or wise. But knowledge and wisdom are really never far away from anyone of us. As a matter of fact, the Bible says that wisdom is everywhere—we just need to open our ears and hear it. The Word of God says, "Wisdom shouts in the streets. She cries out in the public square. She calls out to the crowds along the main street, and to those in front of city hall . . . 'Come here and listen to me! I'll pour out the spirit of wisdom upon you and make you wise'" (Prov. 1:20–21, 23).

Why not simply ask the Lord to give you a wise and understanding heart?

A BIBLE CURE PRAYER
FOR YOU

Dear Lord, open my ears and my mind to Your wisdom. You have given me the precious gift of health. Help me to be a wise and disciplined steward of that wonderful gift. Show me what vitamins and minerals my body may be lacking, and help me to support the natural, God-given sleep that You intended for me to enjoy with the right program of supplements. Amen.

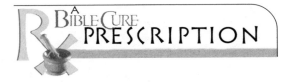

Do you consider your insomnia mild or severe?

_____

I plan to take the following supplements for my
sleep disorder (check boxes):

❑ A good multivitamin/multimineral supplement such as Divine Health Multivitamin

❑ Valerian
Amount: _____

❑ Passionflower
Amount: _____

❑ Hops
Amount: _____

❑ Kava
Amount: _____

❑ St. John's wort
Amount: _____

❑ 5-HTP
Amount: _____

❑ Melatonin
Amount: _____

Chapter 5

Rest Assured
Through Rest in God

How much stress you experience in your daily life does not truly indicate how well you will sleep. One person's life can be full of stress-producing events and situations, and yet this person will be at rest. Another individual's life can be comparatively stress-free, and yet this individual might be filled with tension, turmoil, panic and distress. The difference between the two individuals is not how much stress they encounter, but rather whether or not they are abiding in the vine.

Let me explain. The Bible says, "Remain in me, and I will remain in you. For a branch cannot produce fruit if it is severed from the vine, and you cannot be fruitful apart from me. Yes, I am the vine; you are the branches. Those who remain in me, and I in them, will produce much fruit" (John 15:4–5).

Having peace comes from abiding in Christ. This simply means giving Him all of your anxiety, care and concern and receiving from Him His wisdom, peace, power and love. This wonderful spiritual exchange produces blessed rest in God.

So you can see that what really matters is not the amount of stress in your life but how you actually perceive that stress and react to it. If you react with anger, rage, fear, resentment or any other deadly emotion, you're liable to lose a lot of sleep. But if you react to the stress in your life with faith, trust, peace and reassurance that God is in control, you'll continue to sleep like a baby through every ripple and wave you encounter.

Still, appearances can be deceiving. Sometimes a person who appears calm outwardly can be steaming internally. But it's often difficult to mask your emotions at 2 A.M. when you are lying awake staring at the ceiling. So if you are struggling to get a good night's sleep, your reactions to stress and other deadly emotions may be a key factor.

Therefore, be sure that you're abiding in the vine. Let's examine some important ways of abiding in the vine.

Abiding in the Word of God

Since excessive stress is really all about your perception to the stress, it's critically important to change your perceptions so that they are in line with God's Word. You see, if you truly believe that something can never change, your defeated, hopeless attitude will cause you to feel overwhelmed by stress that robs you of sleep. Therefore, to overcome stress you must learn to take control of your thoughts.

Here are some Bible cure keys: The Word of God says, "Walk in the Spirit, and you shall not fulfill the lust of the flesh" (Gal. 5:16, NKJV). This passage suggests that what you focus upon will empower your thoughts. If you focus upon the Spirit of God through prayer and fill your mind with the Word of God, your thoughts will be filled with the power of God to resist negative, poisonous emotions and attitudes.

Our minds must be renewed so that they will be on the side of the Spirit who is perfect. This renewing of the mind occurs as our thoughts are filled with the powerful, living Word of God. But if our minds are always thinking upon negatives such as what makes us angry, what we don't have that we want, who has hurt us or caused us harm and what we dislike, then our minds and thoughts are carnal or inspired by our lower nature. When we fill our minds with God's words and thoughts through the Bible and prayer, we feed and strengthen our higher nature that was designed to serve God.

This is the secret to overcoming temptation—even the temptation of dangerous emotions. Galatians 5:17 says, "For the flesh lusts against the Spirit, and the Spirit against the flesh; and these are contrary to one another, so that you do not do the things that you wish" (NKJV).

Abiding in Godly Thoughts

If you try and try to push negative, hurtful and destructive carnal thoughts out of your mind, only to find that they return again and again, try this. Meditate on the Word of God by reading these scriptures daily and reflecting upon what they mean.

> Casting down imaginations, and every high thing that exalteth itself against the knowledge of God, and bringing into captivity every thought to the obedience of Christ.
>
> —2 CORINTHIANS 10:5, KJV

Brothers and sisters, think about the things that are good and worthy of praise. Think about the things that are true and honorable and right and pure and beautiful and respected.

—PHILIPPIANS 4:8, NCV

As [a man] he thinketh in his heart, so is he.

—PROVERBS 23:7, KJV

Your attitude should be the same that Christ Jesus had.

—PHILIPPIANS 2:5

Your thoughts, whether godly or carnal, will eventually spill out from your mind and heart in the form of your words. That's why your words are another key for abiding in the vine.

Abiding in Christlike Speech

You've heard that sticks and stones can break your bones but words can never hurt you, right? Well, although it sounds good, nothing could be further from the truth.

What you say has enormous spiritual, emotional and physical power. Proverbs 18:21 says, "Death and life are in the power of the tongue"

(KJV). Your words actually have the power to heal or to kill, to strengthen or to wound, to unite or to divide. Controlling your words is extremely important. Here are some scriptures about the tongue to recite every time you are tempted to slip and say something you know you'll regret:

> Out of the abundance of the heart the mouth speaketh.
>
> —MATTHEW 12:34, KJV

> Every idle word that men shall speak, they shall give an account thereof in the day of judgment.
>
> —MATTHEW 12:36, KJV

> Let no corrupt communication proceed out of your mouth.
>
> —EPHESIANS 4:29, KJV

Abiding in the Power of Forgiveness

One major way to abide in Christlike speech is to make certain that you never harbor hidden grudges, bitterness or anger against anyone. How is such a thing possible in today's hurt-filled world? Only by practicing the power of forgiveness according to Mark 11:25–26: "Whenever you stand praying, if you have anything against anyone, forgive him, that your Father in heaven may also forgive you your trespasses. But if you do not forgive, neither will your Father in heaven forgive your trespasses" (NKJV).

When your soul is washed clean through the power of forgiveness, you will begin to experience a joy that you never before imagined.

Abiding in the Healing Power of Joy

Joy is a deep, peaceful inner happiness that comes from heaven that transcends anything that the world can offer. It is mirth at its highest and peace at its deepest. Only God can give you the power of spiritual joy.

This happiness that comes from heaven has great properties that no carnal, cynical, crude or crass empty laughter ever held. Clean, heavenly joy can actually heal your

> *In thoughts from the visions of the night, when deep sleep falleth on men.*
> —Job 4:13, KJV

body, mind and soul. The Bible says, "A merry heart does good, like medicine" (Prov. 17:22, NKJV). The power of this joy supplies great strength as well. The Bible says, "The joy of the LORD is your strength" (Neh. 8:10, KJV).

You may be wondering, *How can I get this*

heavenly joy? Well, the Bible is quite clear. It says, "In thy presence is fulness of joy" (Ps. 16:11, KJV).

Abiding in God's Love

Why is this supernatural joy so powerful? Well, it's because in this joy you can actually feel and experience the love that God has for you. That's why the last key to abiding in the vine is knowing, understanding and giving to others God's wonderful love.

As you walk in God's love to other people, that love will come back to you, too. The Word of God teaches us, "A new commandment I give you, that you love one another; as I have loved you, that you also love one another. By this all will know that you are My disciples, if you have love for one another" (John 13:34–35, NKJV).

Never forget that love is the greatest commandment of them all.

Understanding and Obeying
the Law of Rest

One of the best ways to overcome the stress in your life is to understand and follow God's law of rest. Let's take a look at this incredible law. The Word of God says, "And six years thou shalt sow thy land,

and shalt gather the fruits thereof: but the seventh year thou shalt let it rest and lie still . . . Six days thou shalt do thy work, and on the seventh day thou shalt rest" (Exod. 23:10–12, KJV).

You can find this same powerful spiritual principle in Exodus 31:15: "Six days may work be done; but in the seventh is the sabbath of rest,

> *For I have given rest to the weary and joy to the sorrowing.*
> —JEREMIAH 31:25

holy to the LORD: whosoever doeth any work in the sabbath day, he shall surely be put to death" (KJV). The next verse goes on to say that this was a perpetual covenant—which means that this principle of Sabbath rest never ends. And verse 17 says, "It is a sign between me and the children of Israel *for ever:* for in six days the LORD made heaven and earth, and on the seventh day he rested, and was refreshed" (KJV, emphasis added).

Today we are not under law, but we live under the grace of God that was purchased for us by Christ Jesus. Nevertheless, rest remains a spiritual principle that we cannot disregard without suffering heavy consequences in terms of our health and well-being.

Although we don't honor the Sabbath by strictly forbidding work on Sundays, we enter into a rest when we learn to depend upon God for everything in our lives. The New Testament talks about this rest when it says, "There remains therefore a Sabbath rest for the people of God" (Heb. 4:9, NAS).

So you can see that rest remains a very present and powerful spiritual principle that God gave to strengthen your body and mind and renew your health and spirit. By honoring the Sabbath rest of God, we rest our bodies and our minds. We refuse to carry around the weight of the daily tension, anxiety, fear and stress of the world. Instead, we let God carry it for us. In doing so, we enter God's rest.

The powerful spiritual principle of God's rest allows our minds and bodies to heal from the effects of stress. The Bible says, "Come to me, all of you who are weary and carry heavy burdens, and I will give you rest" (Matt. 11:28).

In addition, Exodus 15:26 says, "If thou wilt diligently hearken to the voice of the LORD thy God, and wilt do that which is right in his sight, and wilt give ear to his commandments, and keep all his statutes, I will put none of these diseases upon thee, which I have brought upon the Egyptians."

God's rest is a vital key factor in walking in God's divine health for your body, mind and soul.

A BIBLE CURE PRAYER
FOR YOU

Dear Lord, I pray for supernatural rest that refreshes my body, mind, soul and spirit. I choose to take Your yoke. Teach me to know You and to walk in Your wonderful ways. If ever I find myself struggling to enter Your place of rest, I pray beforehand that You meet me at the point of that struggle, and like Jesus rested during the storm, give me inner peace and comfort that I'll make it safely to the other side. Amen.

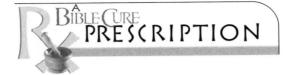

Personalize the following verse of Scripture by filling your own name in the blanks:

The Lord is _____ shepherd; I have everything I need. He lets _____ rest in green meadows; he leads me beside peaceful streams. He renews _____ strength. He guides me along right paths, bringing honor to his name. Even when I walk through the dark valley of death, I will not be afraid, for you are close beside _____. Your rod and your staff protect and comfort me. You prepare a feast for _____ in the presence of my enemies. You welcome _____ as a guest, anointing my head with oil. My cup overflows with blessings. Surely your goodness and unfailing love will pursue _____ all the days of my life, and _____ will live in the house of the Lord forever.

—ADAPTED FROM PSALM 23

A PERSONAL NOTE

From Don and Mary Colbert

God desires to heal you of disease. His Word is full of promises that confirm His love for you and His desire to give you His abundant life. His desire includes more than physical health for you; He wants to make you whole in your mind and spirit as well through a personal relationship with His Son, Jesus Christ.

If you haven't met my best friend, Jesus, I would like to take this opportunity to introduce Him to you. It is very simple.

If you are ready to let Him come into your heart and become your best friend, just bow your head and sincerely pray this prayer from your heart:

Lord Jesus, I want to know You as my Savior and Lord. I believe You are the Son of God and that You died for my sins. I also believe You were raised from the dead and now sit at the right hand of the Father praying for me. I ask You to forgive me for my sins and change my heart so that I can

be Your child and live with You eternally.
Thank You for Your peace. Help me to
walk with You so that I can begin to know
You as my best friend and my Lord. Amen.

If you have prayed this prayer, we rejoice with you in your decision and your new relationship with Jesus. Please contact us at pray4me@strang.com so that we can send you some materials that will help you become established in your relationship with the Lord. You have just made the most important decision of your life. We look forward to hearing from you.

Notes

PREFACE
REST ASSURED

1. "2000 Omnibus Sleep in America Poll," National Sleep Foundation, 1522 K Street NW, Suite 500, Washington, DC.
2. Ibid.

CHAPTER 1
REST ASSURED—YOU CAN FIND REST!

1. *Good Night America: Deep Sleep Reference Guide* (n.p.: Good Night America L.L.C., 1998), 26.

CHAPTER 3
REST ASSURED THROUGH EXERCISE AND LIFESTYLE CHANGES

1. M. Scofield, *Worksite Health Promotion* (Philadelphia: Hanley and Belfus, 1990), 459.
2. Hans Selye, *The Stress of Life* (New York: McGraw-Hill, 1956).
3. W. F. Waters et al., "Attention, Stress and Negative Emotion and Persistent Sleep-Onset and Sleep-Maintenance Insomnia," *Sleep* 16:2 (1993): 128–136.
4. Joseph Pizzorno and Michael Murray, *Textbook of Natural Medicine* (New York: Churchill Livingstone, 1999), 546.
5. For more information about full spectrum lights or light boxes, call the Sun Box Company at 1-800-LITE-YOU or Environmental Lighting Concepts, Inc. at 1-800-842-8848.
6. Personalized Sleep Plan Checklist, *Good Night America: Deep Sleep Reference Guide.*

CHAPTER 4
REST ASSURED THROUGH SUPPLEMENTS

1. P. D. Leathwood et al., "Aqueous Extract of Valerian Root Improves Sleep Quality in Man," *Pharmacol Biochem Behav* 17 (1982): 65–71.
2. H. P. Volz et al., "Kava-kava Extract WS 1490 Versus Placebo in Anxiety Disorders," *Pharmacopsychiatry* 30(1) (1997): 1–5.

Don Colbert, M.D., was born in Tupelo, Mississippi. He attended Oral Roberts School of Medicine in Tulsa, Oklahoma, where he received a bachelor of science degree in biology in addition to his degree in medicine. Dr. Colbert completed his internship and residency with Florida Hospital in Orlando, Florida. He is board certified in family practice and has received extensive training in nutritional medicine.

If you would like more
information about natural and
divine healing, or information about
Divine Health Nutritional Products®,
you may contact
Dr. Colbert at:

Dr. Don Colbert

1908 Boothe Circle
Longwood, FL 32750
Telephone: 407-331-7007

Dr. Colbert's website is
www.drcolbert.com.

Announcing